**This Book
Belongs To:** _____

www.powerbookbags.org

100 SOUNDS TO SEE

Marsha Engle

William J. Huber
Photographer

Health Communications, Inc.
Deerfield Beach, Florida

www.hcibooks.com

Library of Congress Cataloging-in-Publication Data

Engle, Marsha.

  100 sounds to see / Marsha Engle ; William Huber, photographer.

    p.   cm.

  ISBN-13: 978-0-7573-1538-1

  ISBN-10: 0-7573-1538-0

  1. Sounds. 2. Sounds—Pictorial works. 3. Hearing. I. Huber, William. II. Title. III. Title: One hundred sounds to see.   IV. Title: Hundred sounds to see.

  QC225.3.E54 2010

  617.8'0651—dc22

2010015707

Publisher: Health Communications, Inc.
        3201 S.W. 15th Street
        Deerfield Beach, FL 33442–8190

Photography ©William Huber
Cover and interior formatting by Lawna Patterson Oldfield

For every book sold, Marsha Engle will donate a portion of her proceeds to the
American Academy of Audiology Foundation to support pediatric audiology research.

*I*t was supposed to be just for me. As my world was growing softer by the year, I wanted something that would help me to remember them all . . . the sounds of an ordinary day.

William Huber is an extraordinary photographer and he agreed to help me in my quest to capture pictures of the sounds I could no longer hear. Perhaps if I had something to trigger the memory by sight, I could somehow keep those sounds safely tucked away in my mind.

What happened was something much more powerful, more meaningful, and useful to many; it was no longer just for me. It comes in the form of a collection of 100 beautiful photographs of sounds . . . sounds I wish I could hear. The end result is a treasure that reminds us of this important life lesson: what is so normal is really quite profound.

So, hearing world, I want to share with you my gift from William. *100 Sounds to See* is a tool that will teach you to first notice and then listen to the sounds of your day. Really listen. In this world of stress, fear, and anxiety, it was there for you all along . . . a free ticket to inner peace, no matter what the world throws your way.

What I miss the most doesn't come from an MP3 player, a cell phone, or anything technical. The sounds aren't the stuff of concertos or marching bands. They are often subtle, soft, and easy to miss. But they are so rich and so nurturing, and they are yours.

I loved them all, these sounds. Now I ask you to listen to your world. Even just for a few moments, listen to your life.

—Marsha

During the Day

Let the rain kiss you.

Let the rain beat upon your head with silver liquid drops.

Let the rain sing you a lullaby.   Langston Hughes

The *drip* of thawing ice

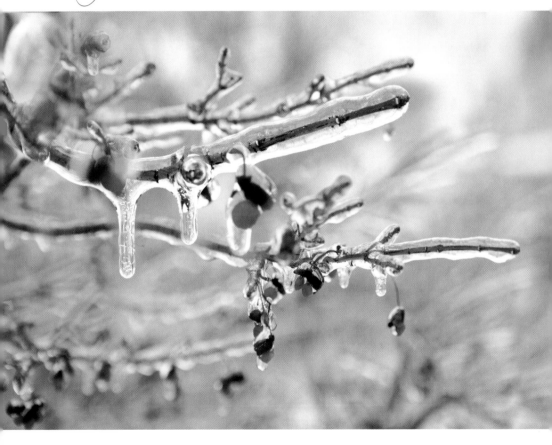

The *hiss* of a radiator

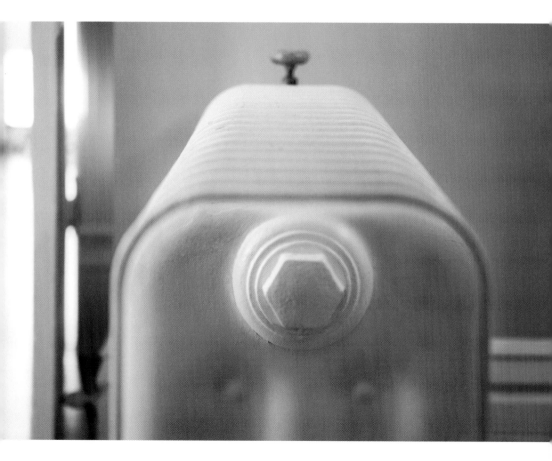

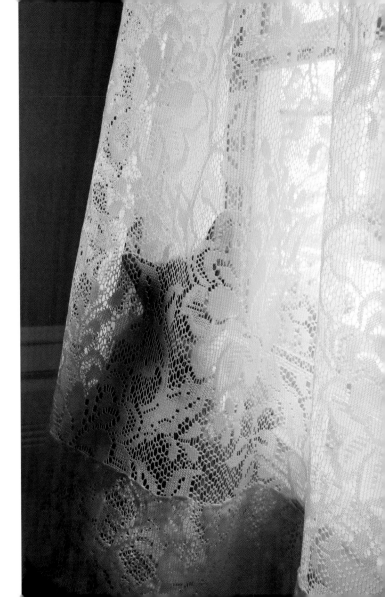

A

curious

cat's

purr

The *rumbling* of an approaching storm

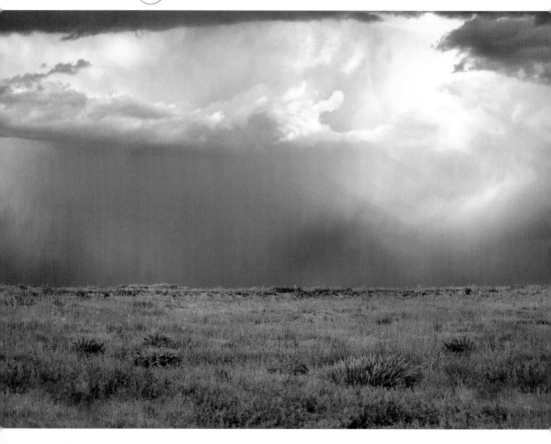

The skate's *scrape* on a frozen pond

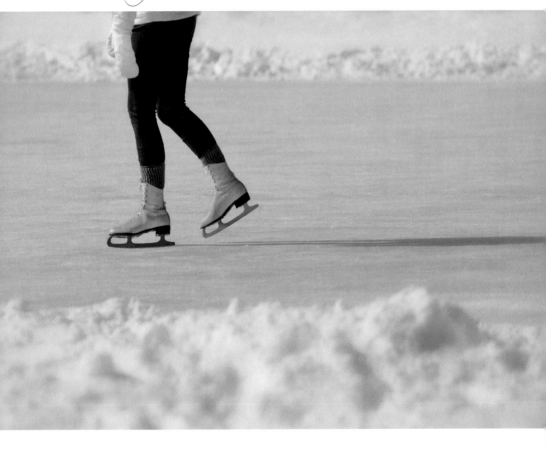

A pot of fresh coffee *perking*

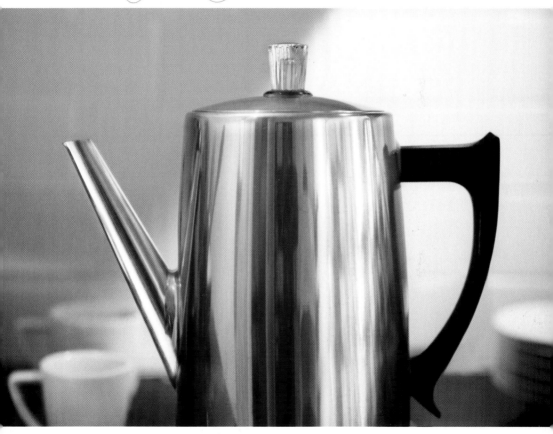

A persistent squirrel's *chatter*

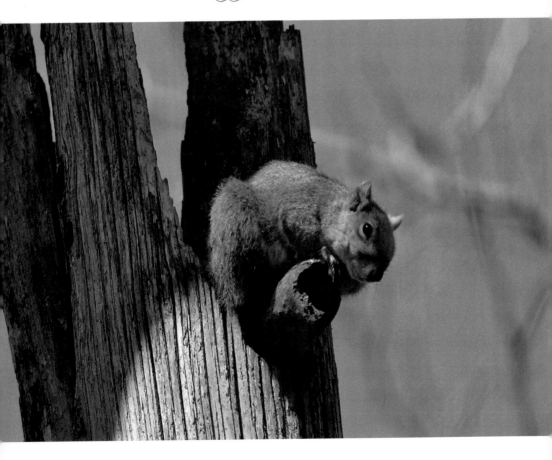

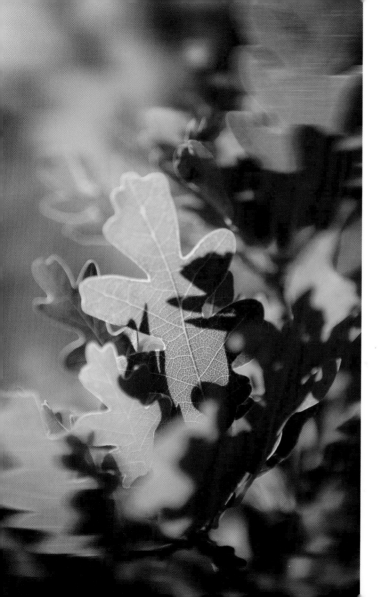

The

rustle

of oak leaves

in the wind

The *spray* of a sod sprinkler

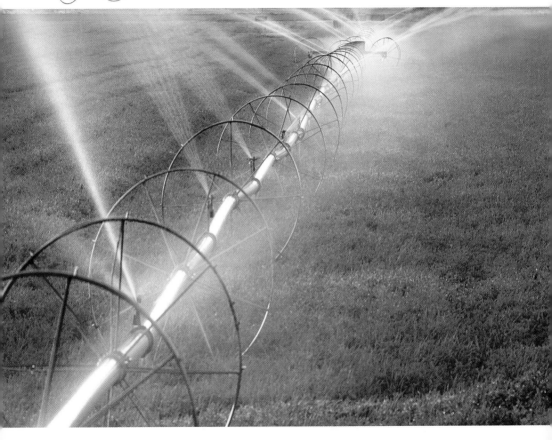

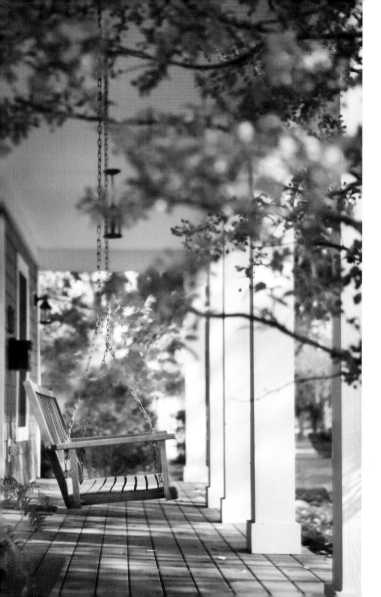

The

creak

of a

porch

swing

Freshly laundered sheets *flapping* on a clothesline

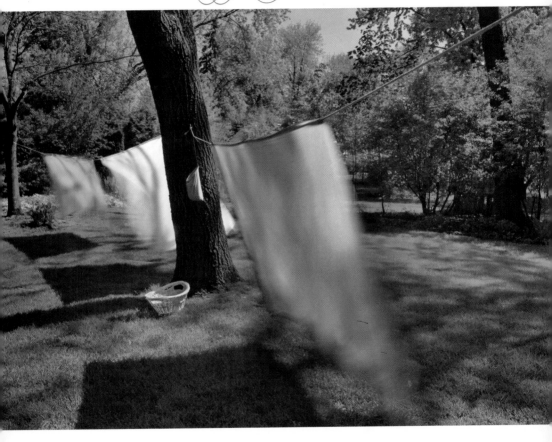

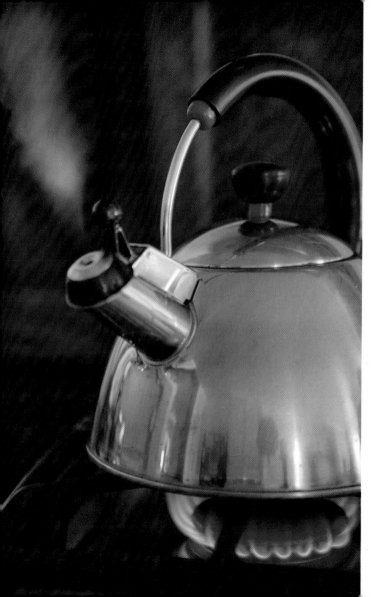

The

whistling

of a

tea kettle

A ball *bouncing*

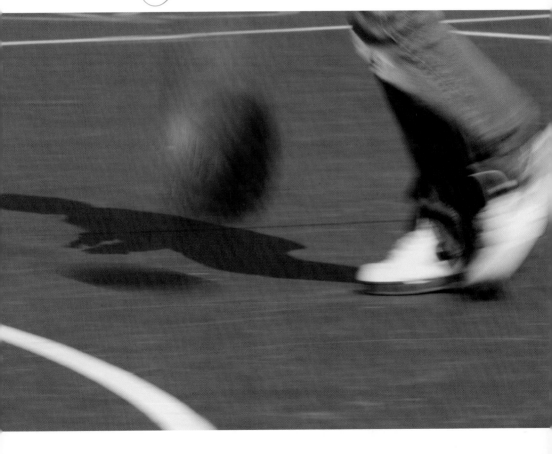

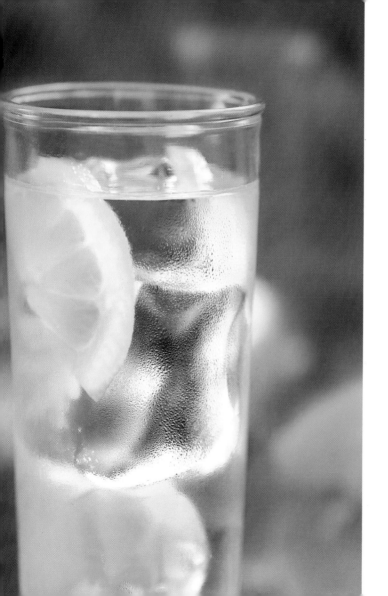

Ice

crackling

in a

glass of

lemonade

Cereal *pouring* into a bowl

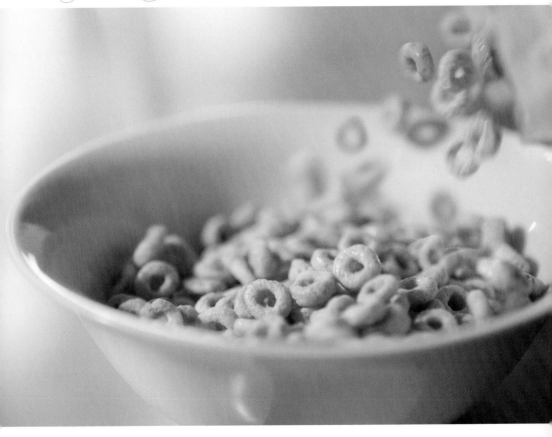

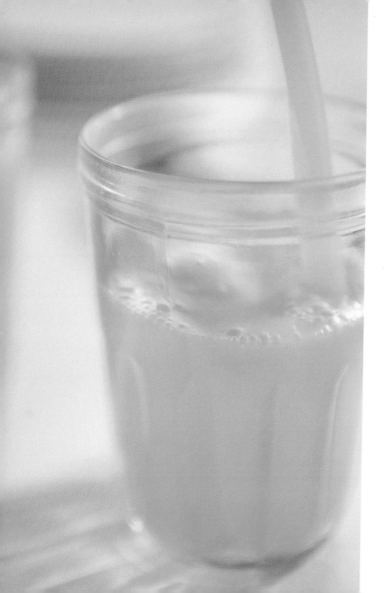

Juice

sloshing

into a

glass

The *turning* spokes of a bicycle

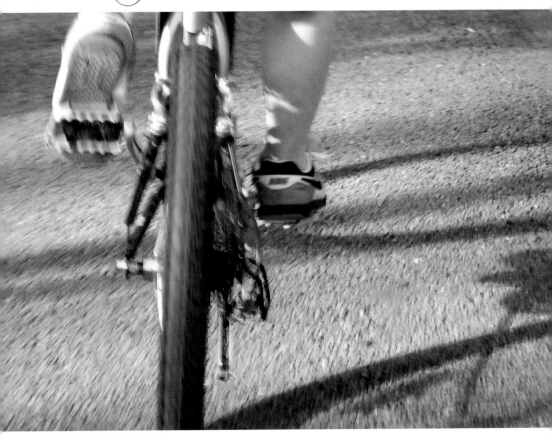

The *stream* of a morning shower

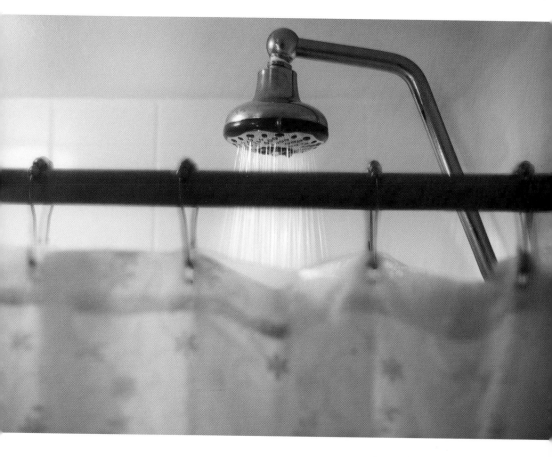

The

buzz

of bees

in a

garden

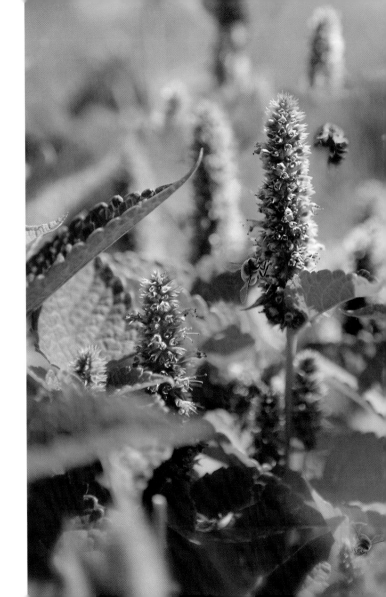

Bacon *sizzling* in a pan

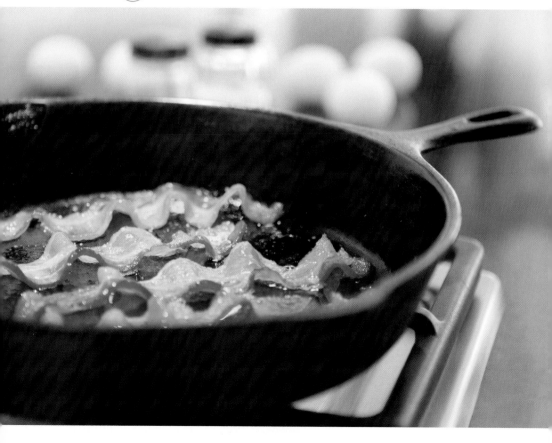

The

scrunch

of buttering

toast

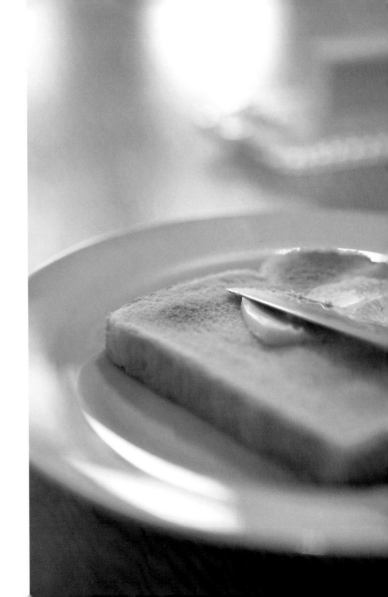

The *pounding* feet of a jogger

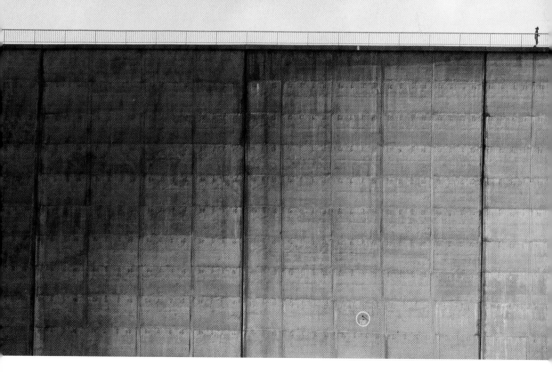

A spring bird's *chirp*

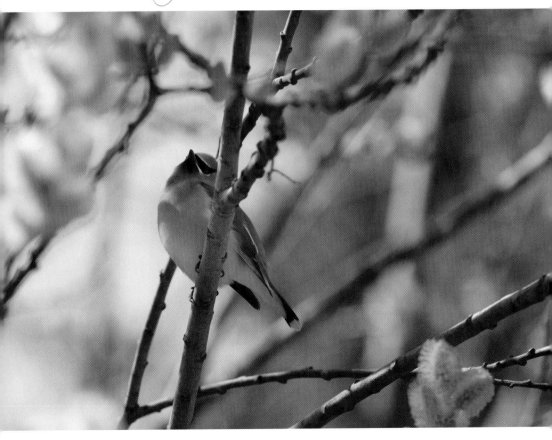

Rain *pattering* on the roof

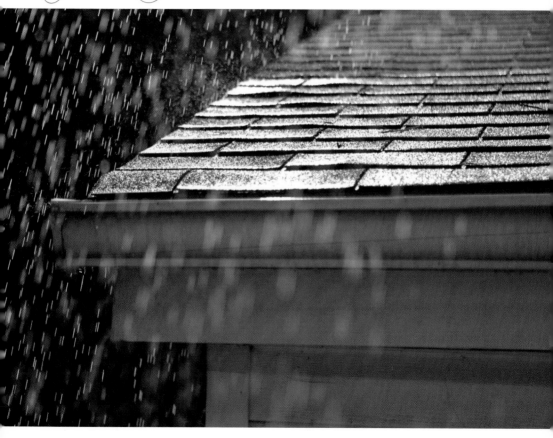

The

whir

of a

fan

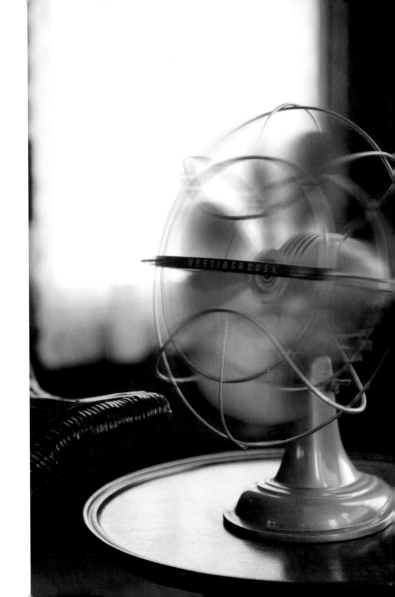

Through the Night

I t takes solitude under the stars, for us to be reminded of our eternal origin and our far destiny.   ARCHIBALD RUTLEDGE

The

whirl

of

carnival

rides

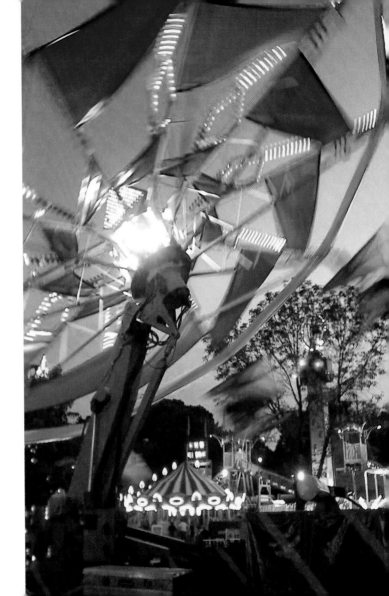

The *snapping* flames of a campfire

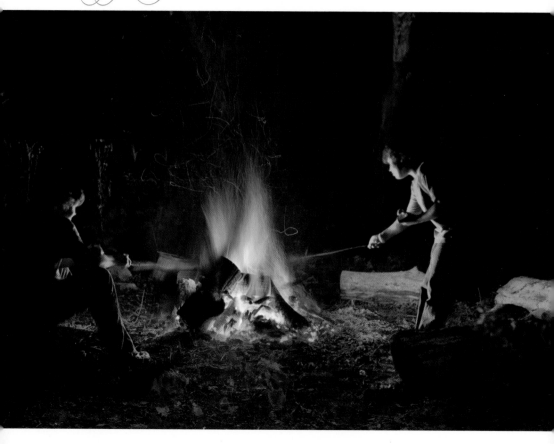

A

grandfather

clock

ticking

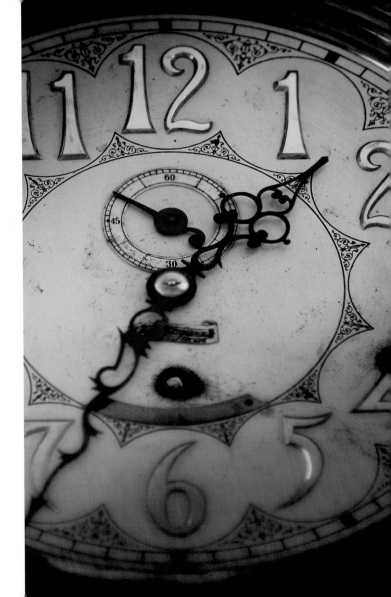

The distant 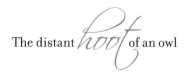 of an owl

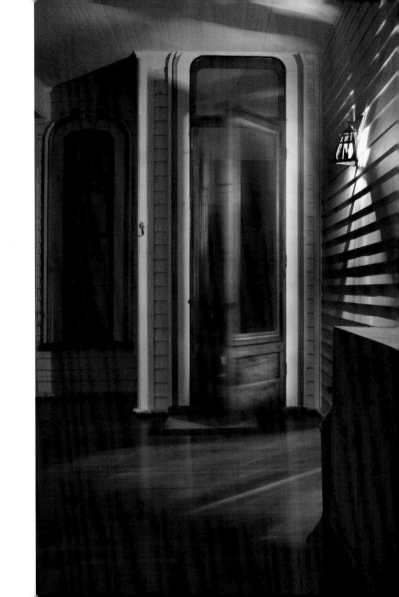

The

slam

of a

screen

door

The *turn* of a page

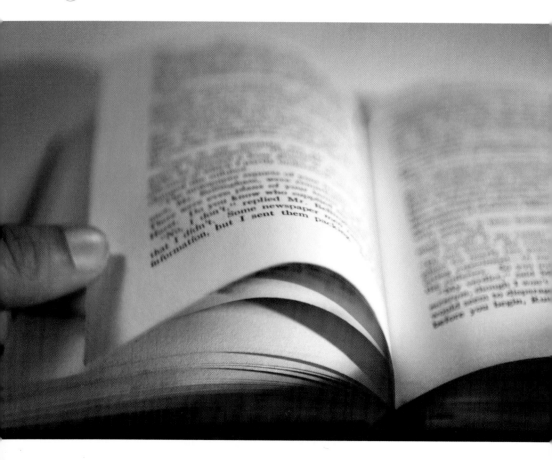

The

strike

of a

match

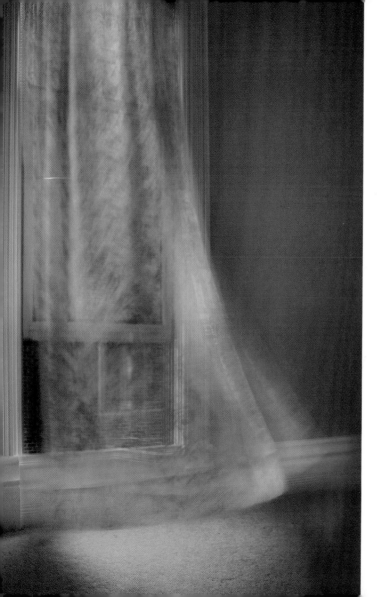

A curtain

blowing

against

a screen

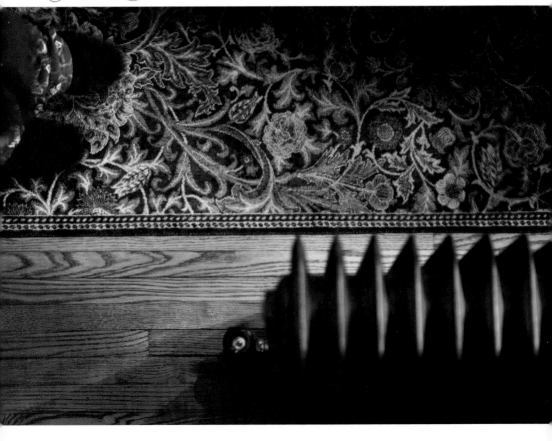

The *padding* of slippers

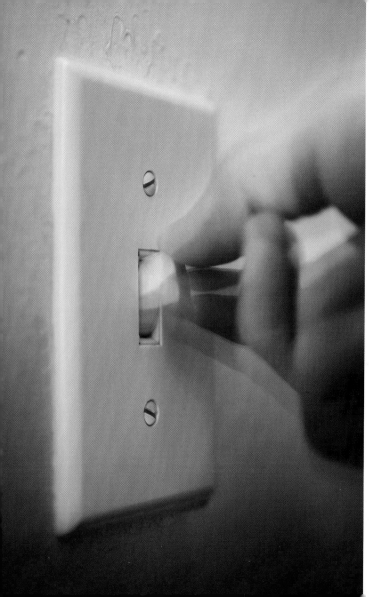

The

flip
of a
switch

The *giggles* of children

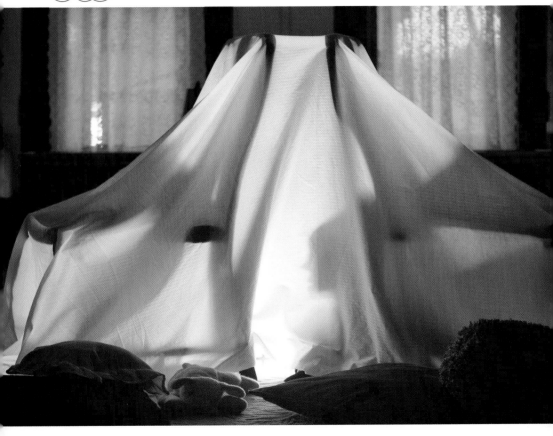

Frogs *croaking* in a pond

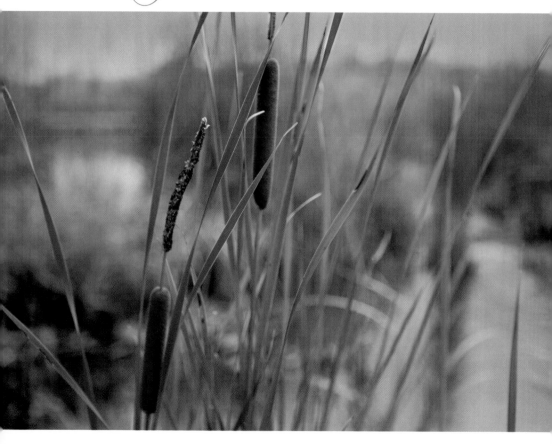

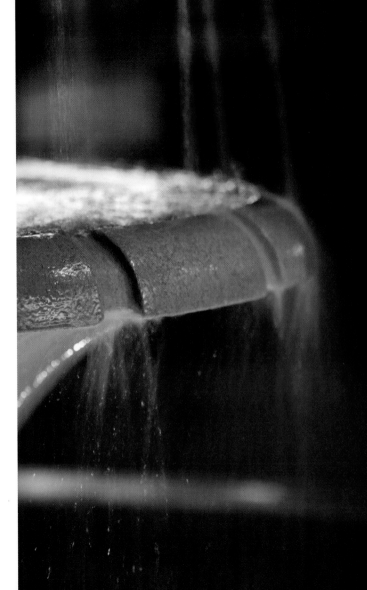

Water *splashing* in a fountain

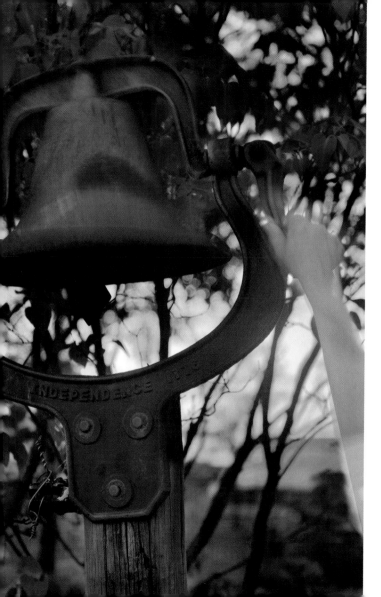

The

clang

of a

dinner

bell

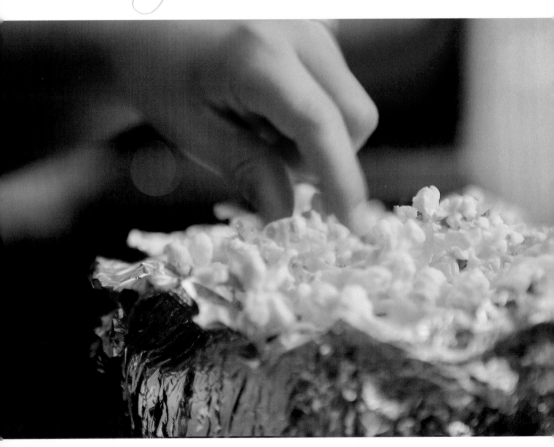

Munching on popcorn

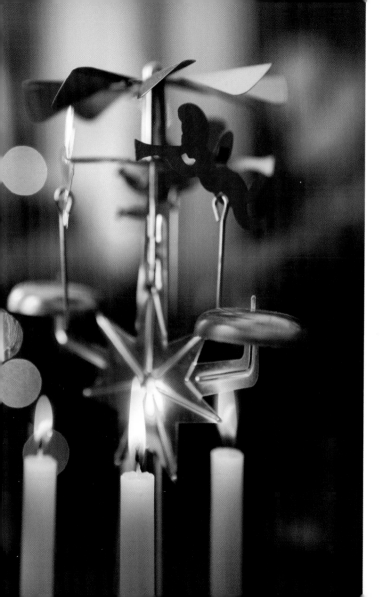

The

delicate

tingle

of angel

chimes

The

one-note

song of

a train

whistle

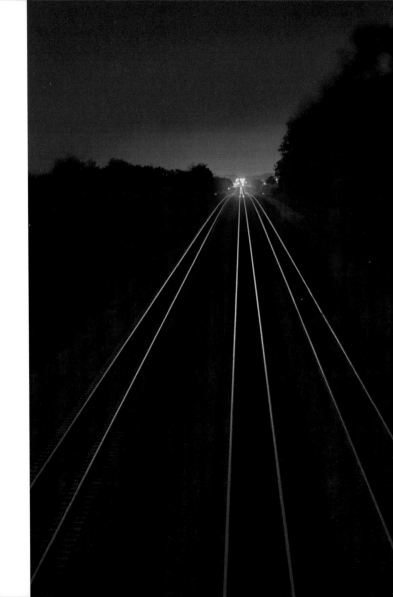

An alarm clock *beeping*

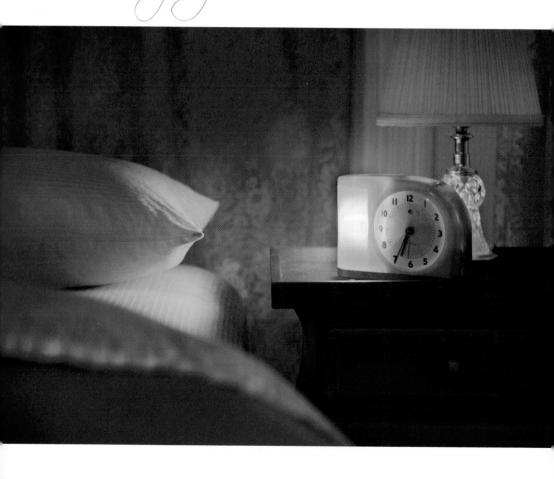

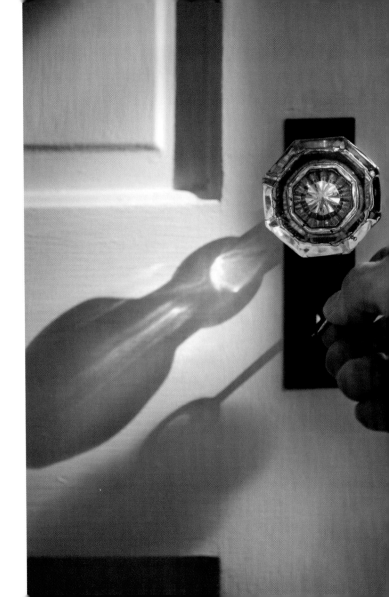

The

click

of a

lock

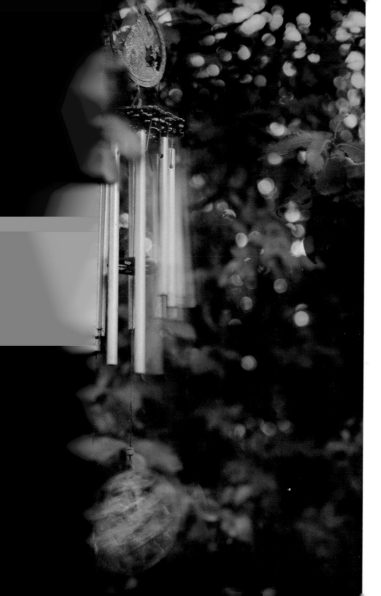

Wind

chimes

tinkling

The

trickle

of a

creek

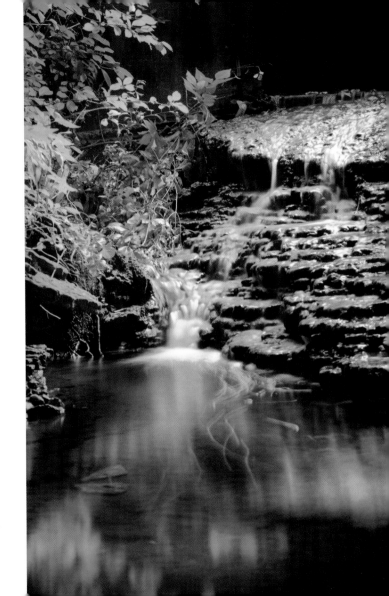

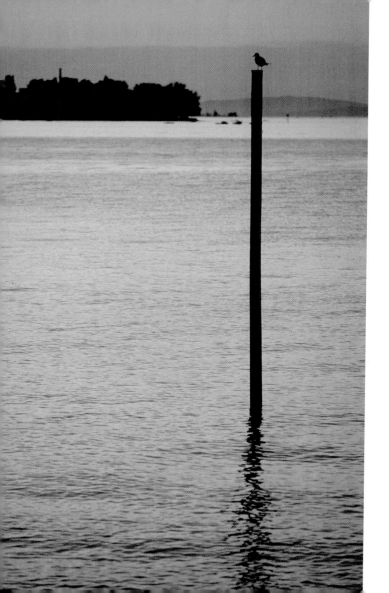

A lake's
gentle *lap*
against
a piling

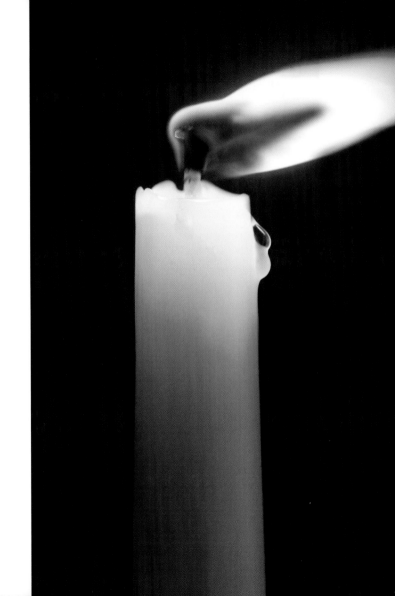

Blowing
out a
candle

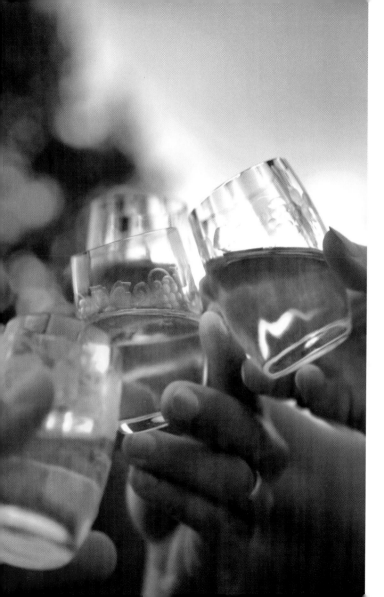

The

clink

of a

toast

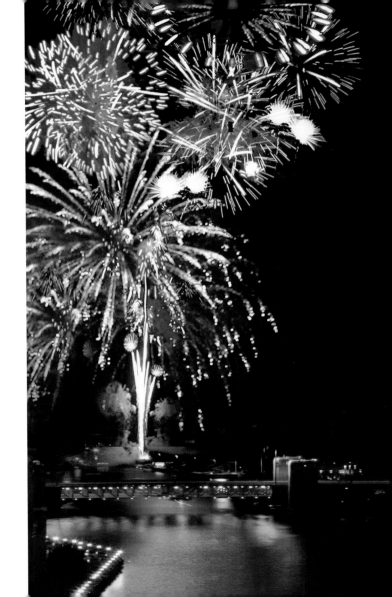

The

booming

of a

fireworks

finale

Places Near & Far

The everyday kindness of the back roads more than makes up for the agony of the headlines. CHARLES KURALT

The *thwack* of a bat at the ballpark

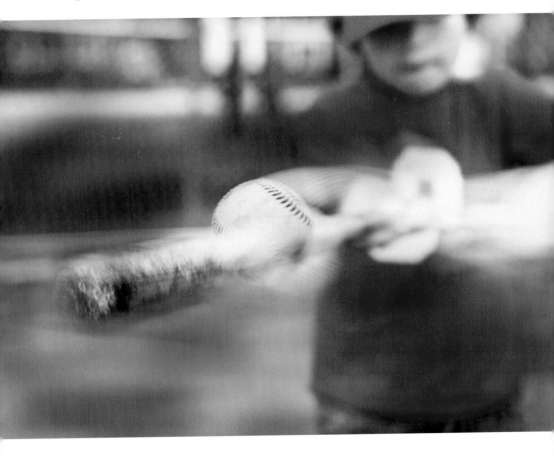

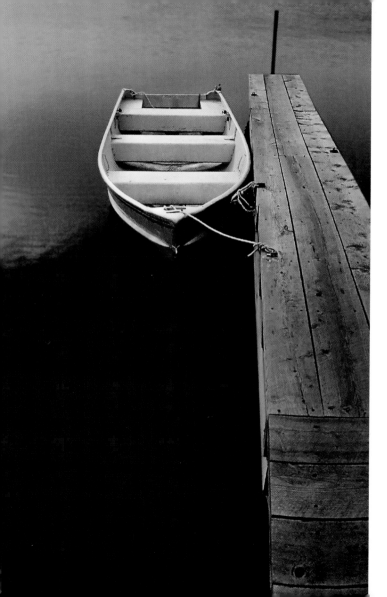

A rowboat

knocking

against

the dock

The *churn* of a river

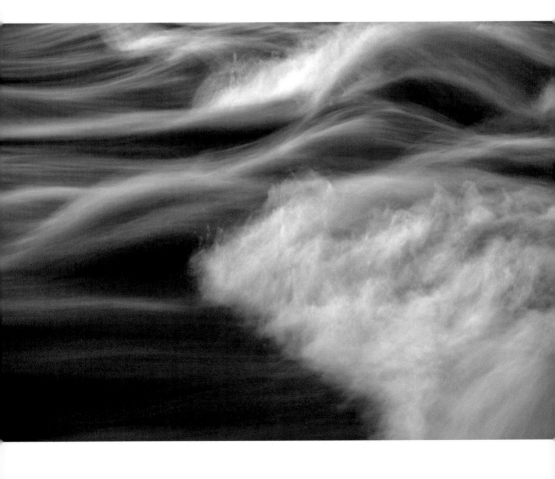

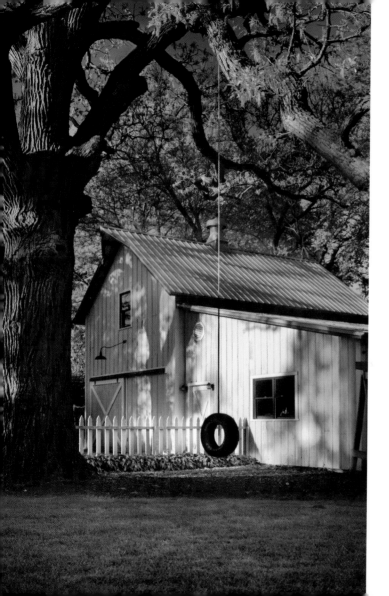

The

whoosh

of a

tire swing

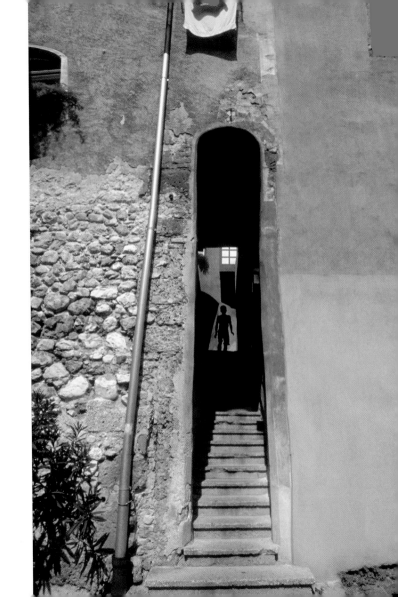

Footsteps

on stone

stairs

A *humming* bird in the garden

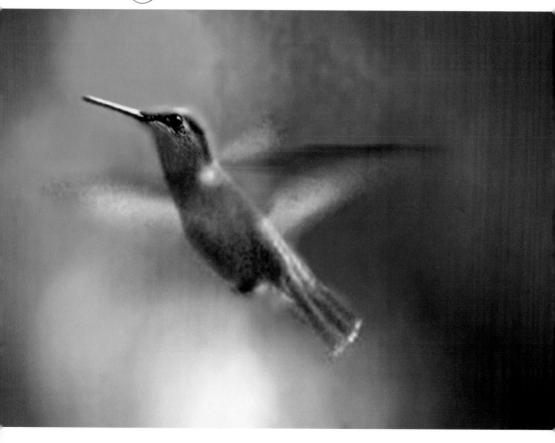

A brisk *breeze* through the cherry blossoms

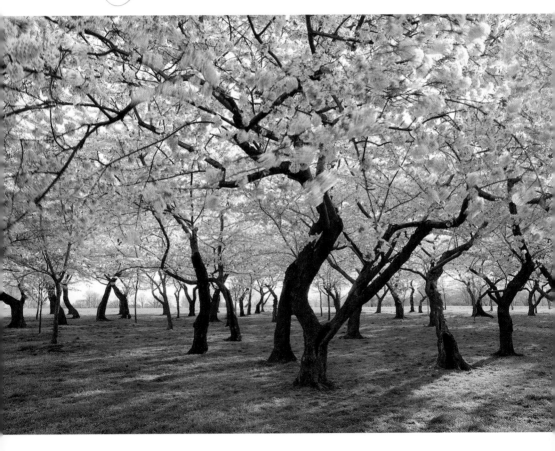

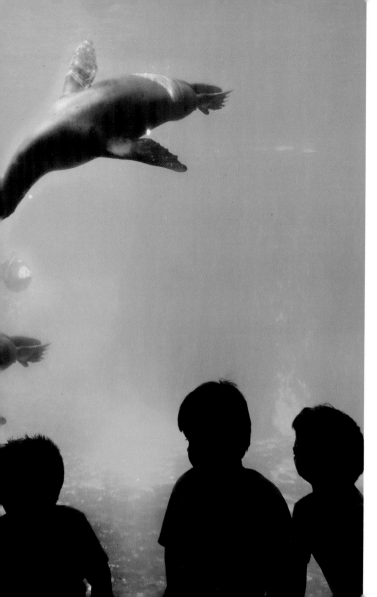

Hushed

voices at an

aquarium

Birds *gathering* on a telephone wire

A dousing *splash* at the water park

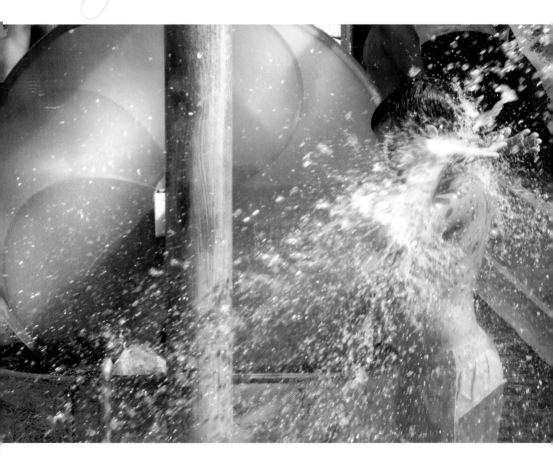

Waves *crashing* by a lighthouse

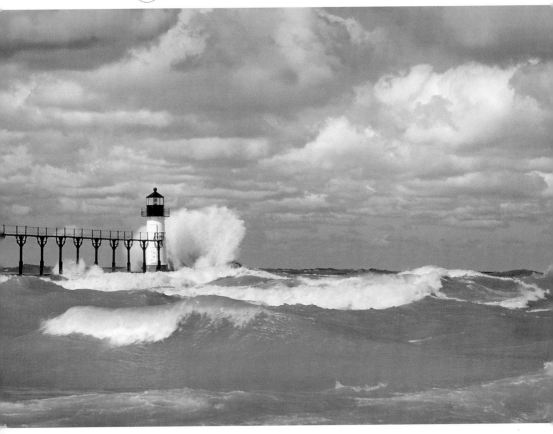

Chickens *clucking* in a barn

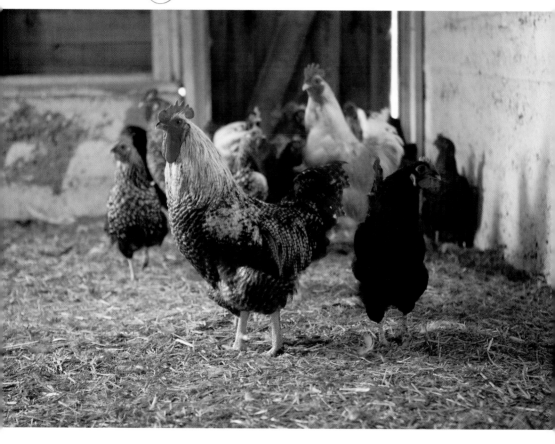

The *bustle* of a farmer's market

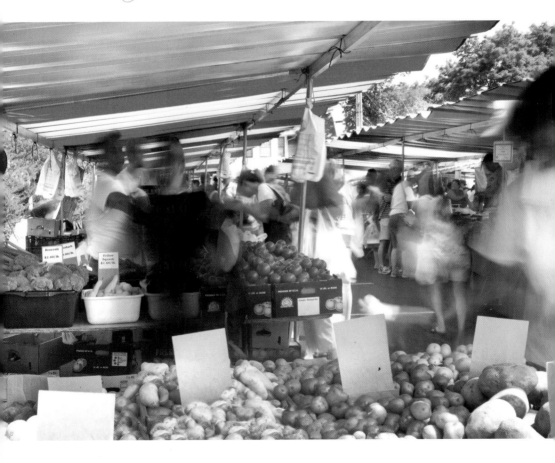

The *chug* of a tractor through the field

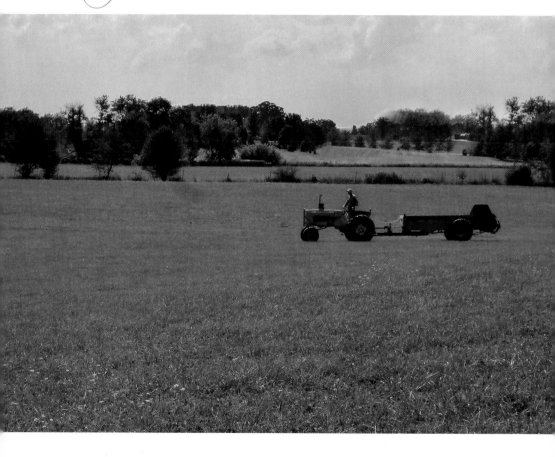

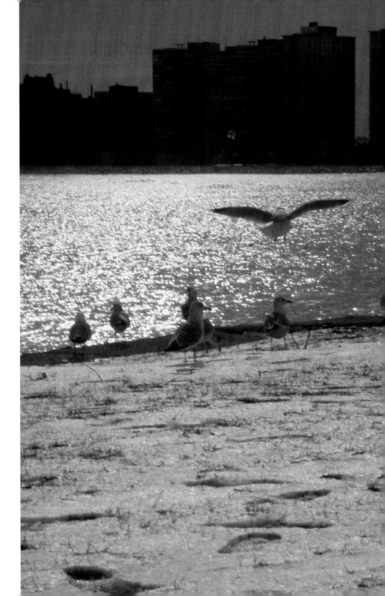

The

cries

of seagulls

by a

shoreline

Wind *stirring* a field of flowers

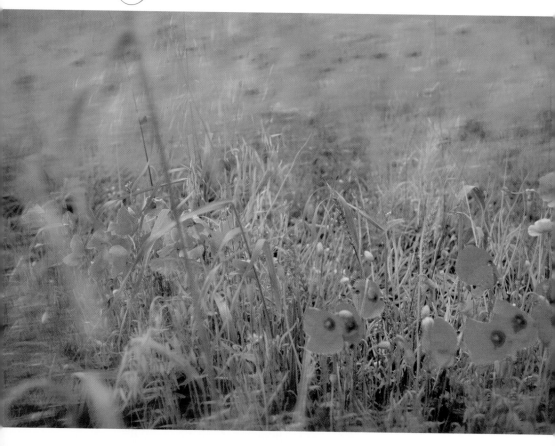

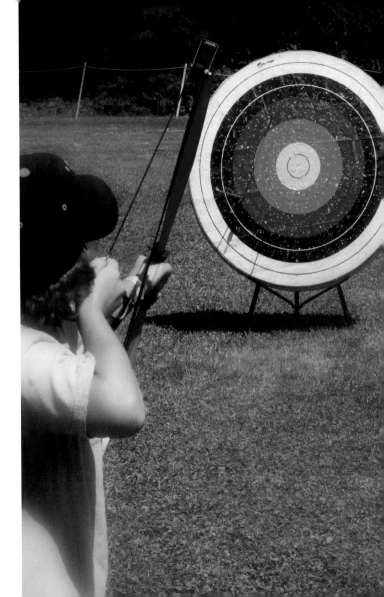

The

swish

of an arrow

at the

range

The *wash* of an incoming tide

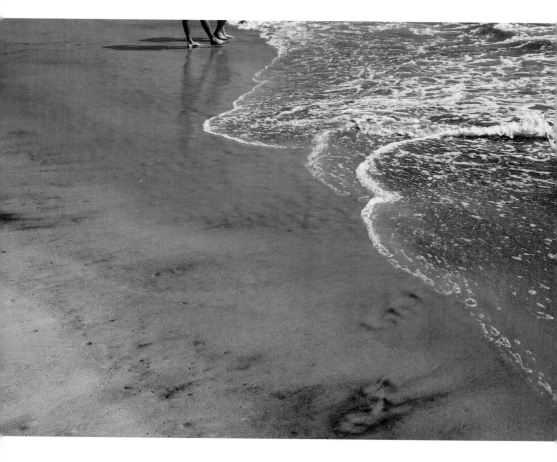

The *drone* of crowds at a beach

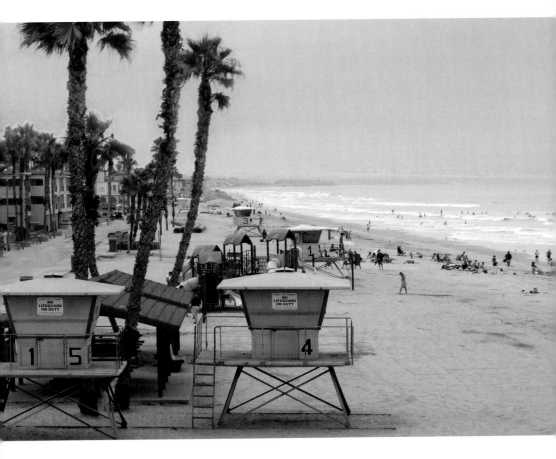

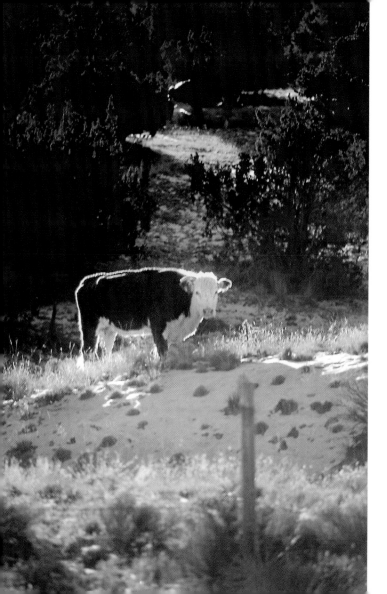

A cow

mooing

in the

field

The *crunch* of ice on a river's edge

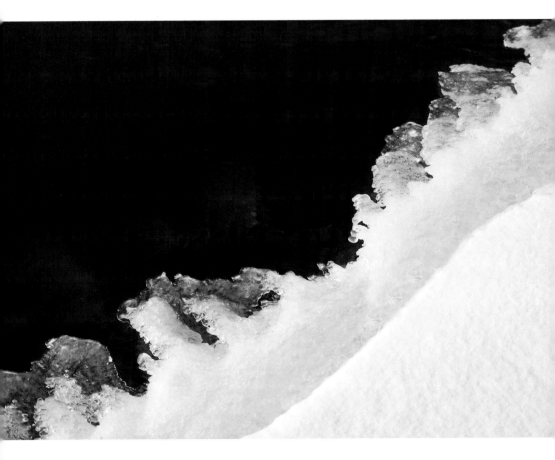

Bells *chiming* in the steeple

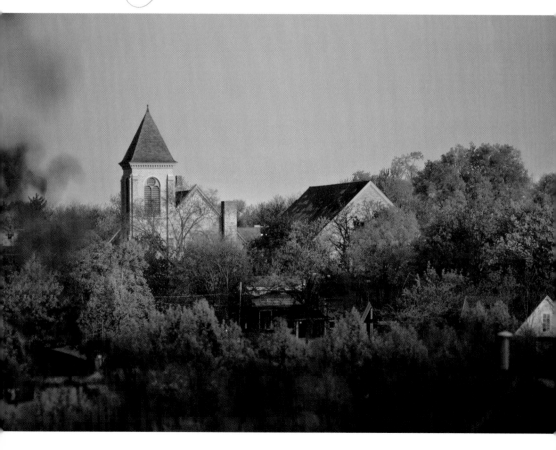

A horse *grazing* in the pasture

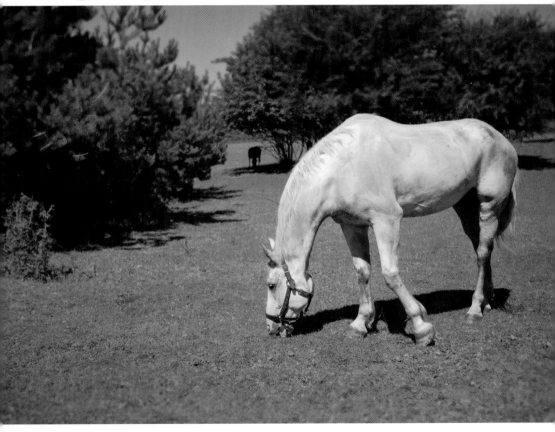

The *rush* of a waterfall

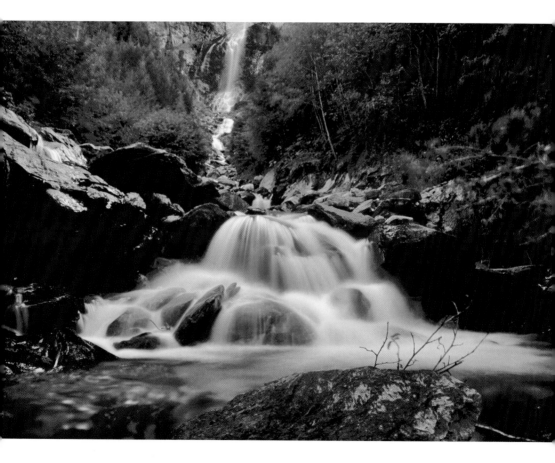

The *grinding* of a gravel road

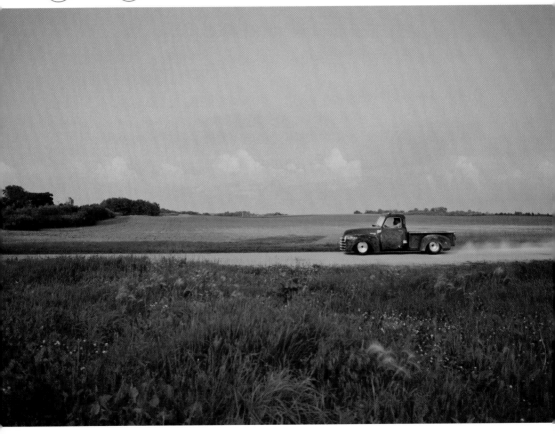

Moments in Life

*J*ust put your ear down next to your soul and listen hard.   ANNE SEXTON

Planes

zooming

overhead

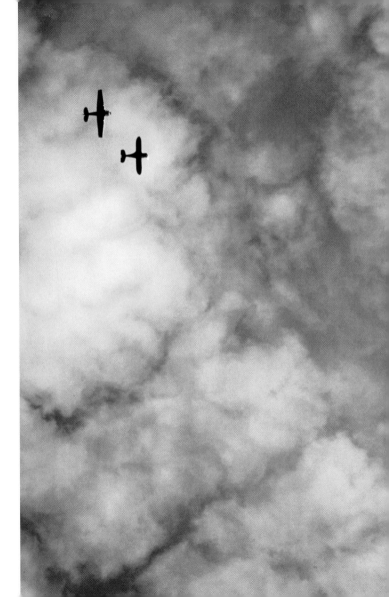

A wet dog *shaking*

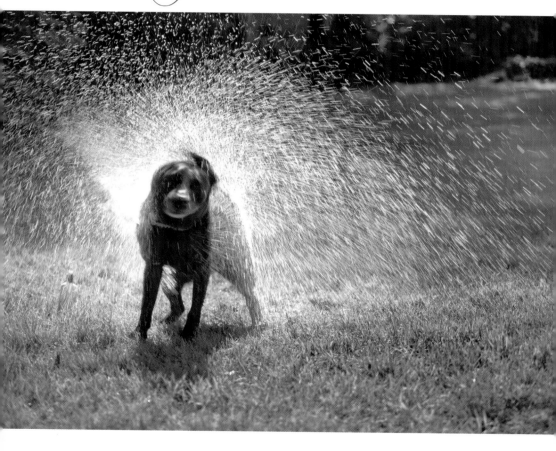

The *crunch* of an apple

The *shhhh* of a conch shell

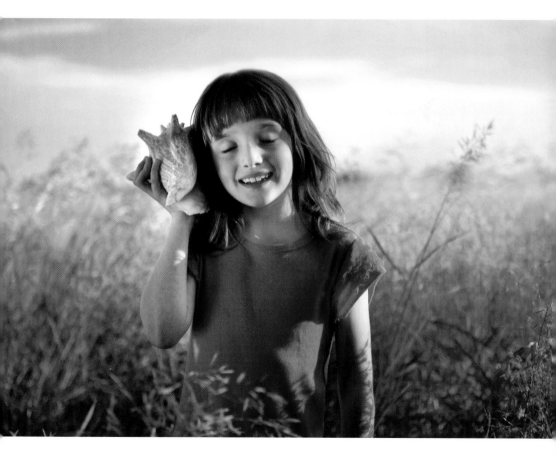

A baby's *laugh*

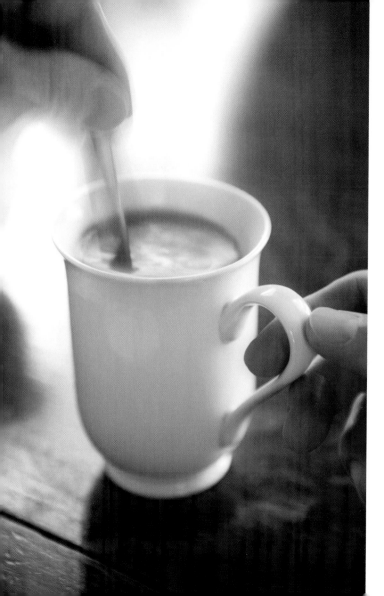

A

ting

of the

spoon in

a cup

The *snap* of a green bean

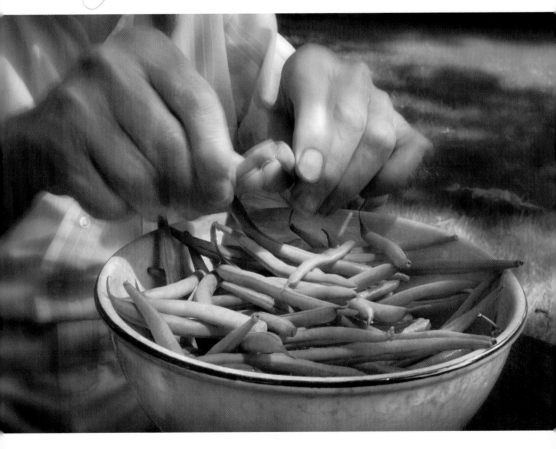

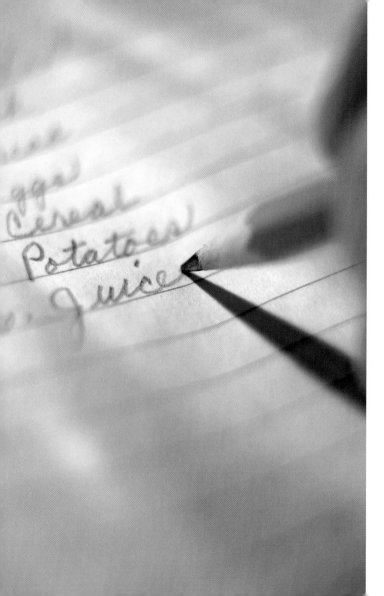

The

scratch

of a

pencil

The *tap* of fingers on piano keys

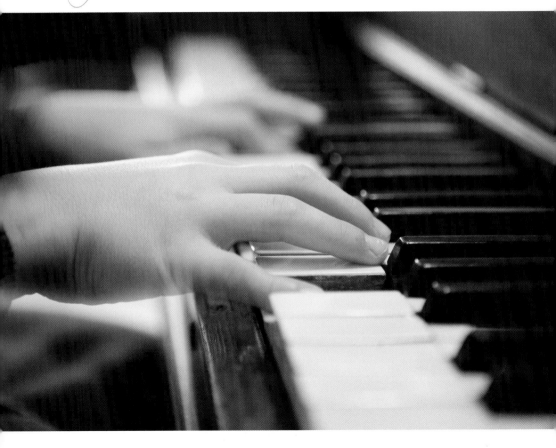

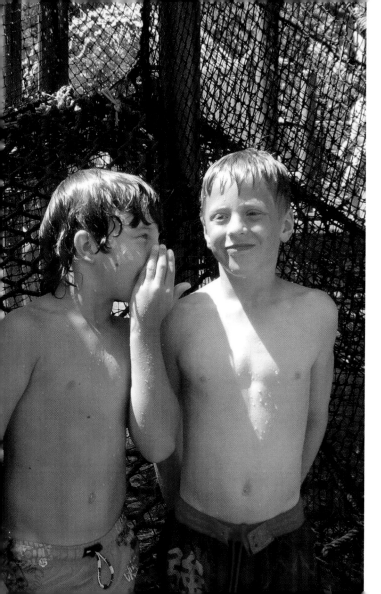

A

whispered

secret

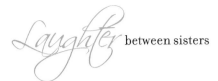

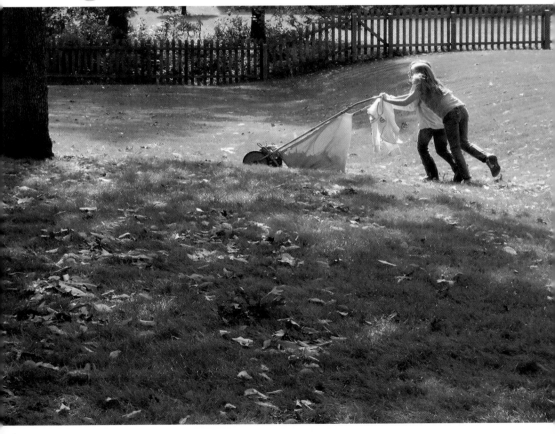

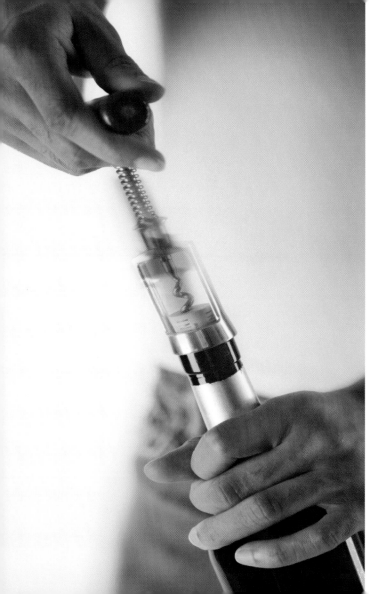

A

pop

of the

cork

The *crack* of a walnut

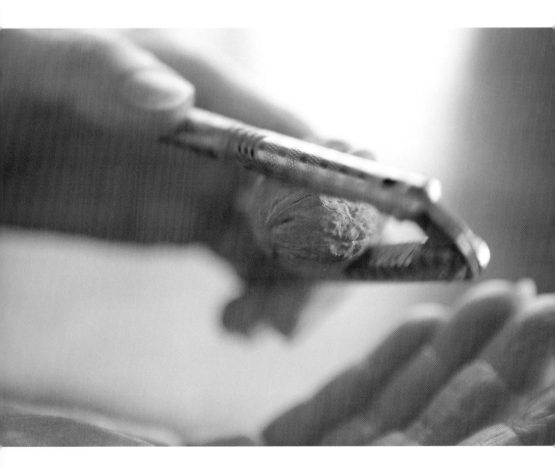

The *squeak* of a teeter-totter

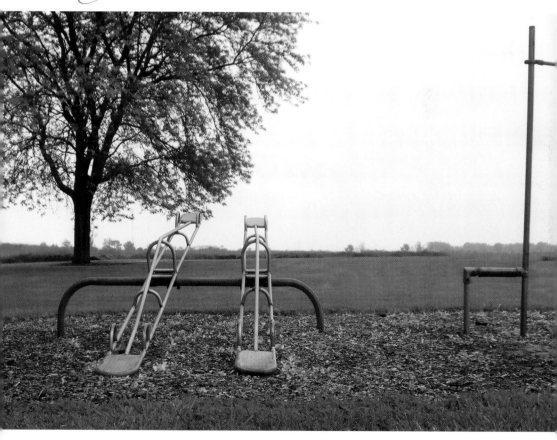

The

swipe

of a

squeegee

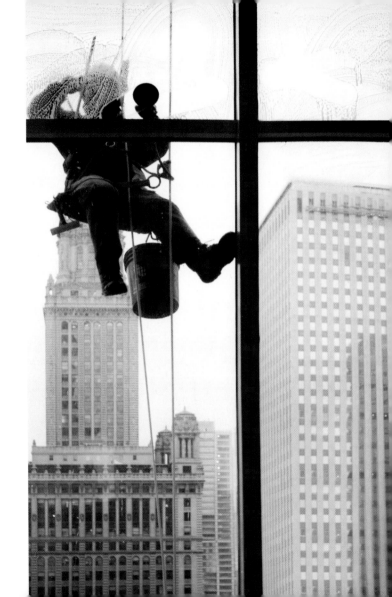

Newborn birds *peeping* in their nest

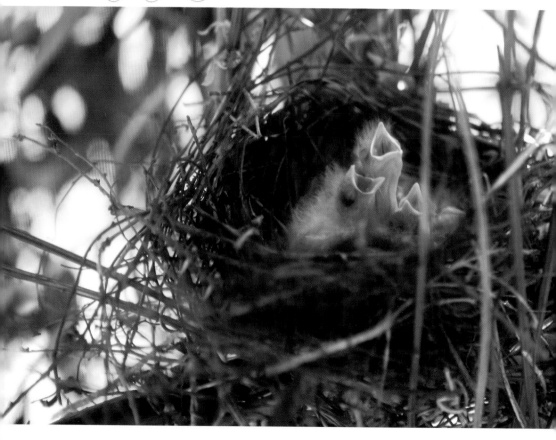

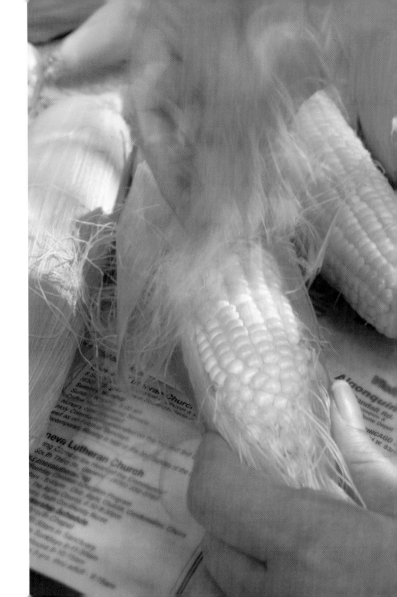

The

shuck

of a husk

of corn

The flag *unfurling* in a breeze

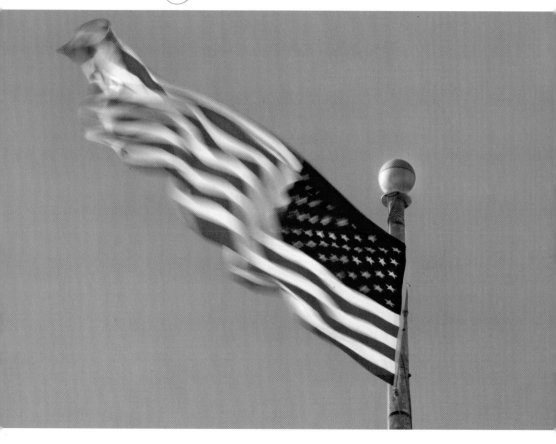

The *ringing* of an incoming call

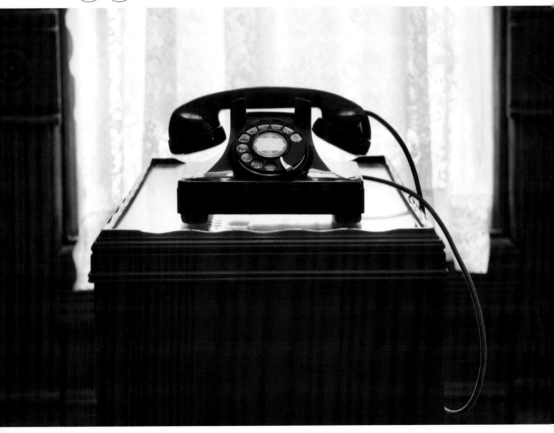

The leisurely *conversation* of teenagers

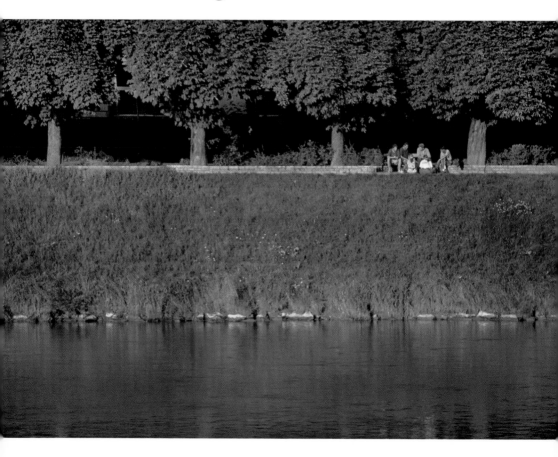

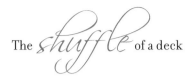
The *shuffle* of a deck

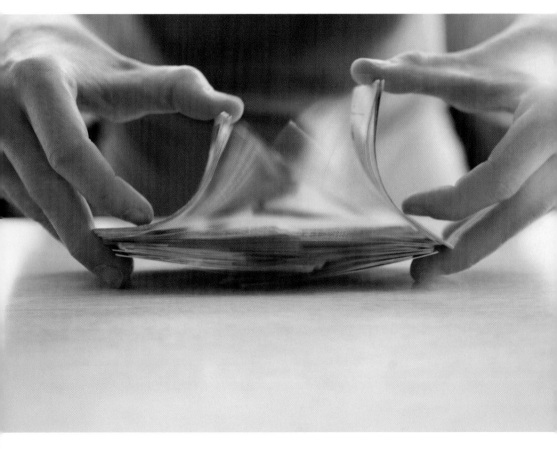

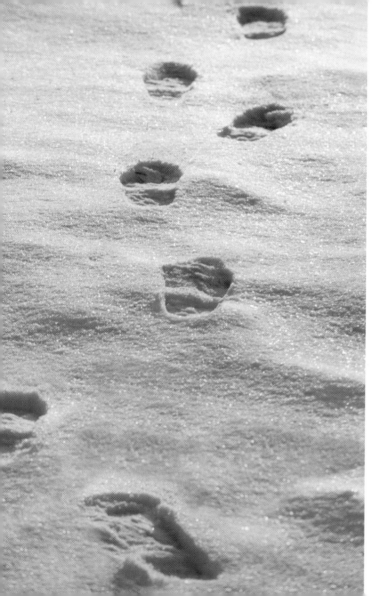

Snow

crunching

underfoot

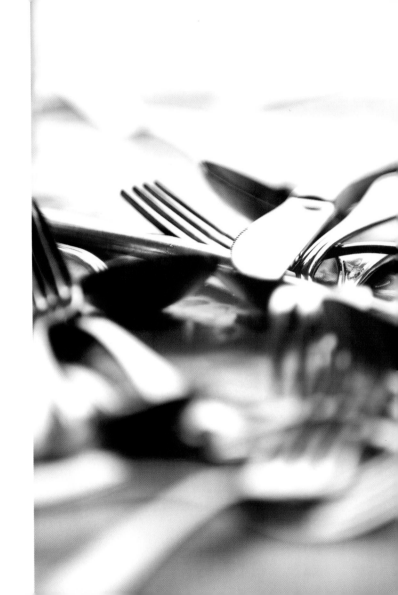

The
clang
of
sivlerware

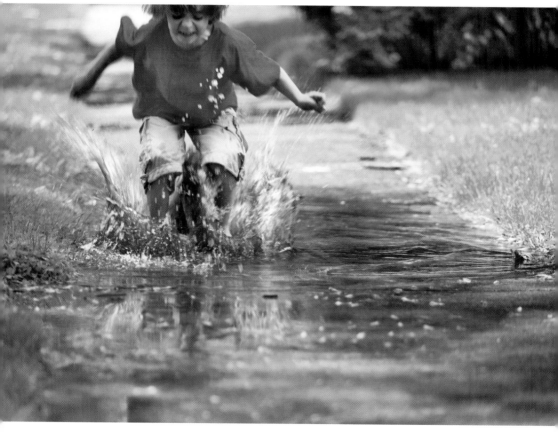

A *splash* in a puddle

The 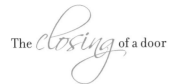 of a door

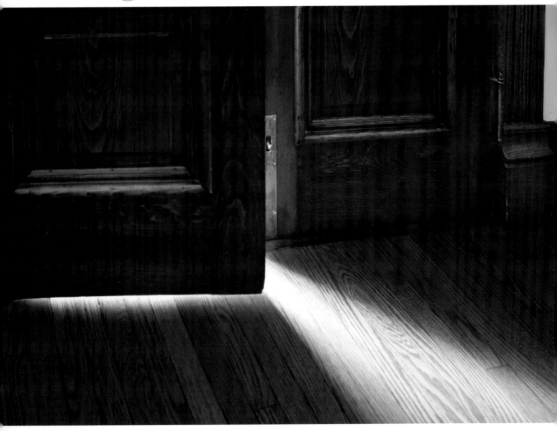

Acknowledgments

*T*hank you to Bill Huber. Your passion, along with your artistic brilliance, is what made this book a reality.

Thank you to Mary Beth Janssen, my author coach and mentor.

To Michael Santucci, you have given me the tools to be a part of the hearing world for more years than we will count.

To my agent, Kristina Holmes, thank you for believing that there was a home for this book.

To my editor at HCI Books, Carol Rosenberg, for giving this book a home.

To Bill Paetzold, your design input and literary expertise is so appreciated.

And finally, thank you to all my family and friends for endless patience. No matter how many times you had to repeat yourselves . . . you always made me feel included.

About the Author

Marsha Engle has been hearing impaired since childhood due to a progressive sensory neural loss. Now legally deaf, Marsha leads a relatively normal life through hearing aids and skilled lip reading. While the sounds of an ordinary day have slowly disappeared, Marsha was inspired to create this book to remind the rest of us that the everyday sounds of life are to be treasured. Marsha lives in Geneva, Illinois, with her husband, Mark; daughter, Gracie; and loyal canine hearing assistant, Mickey.

About the Photographer

William J. Huber sees extraordinary images in ordinary sights. He creates art that showcases subjects from a unique perspective for clients in North America and Europe. His personal passion is traveling the long, winding miles of old road "Route 66" with his son Nathan, visually documenting the imagery of vanishing everyday Americana. For more information, visit www.huberphotography.com.

Visit www.100soundstosee.com and https://100soundstosee.blogspot.com and become a fan on Facebook!